Survival Medicine:

Learn How To Heal Yourself At Home Or In The Wilderness + Herbal Antibiotics Guide

Table of content

Book 1

Adam Bell

SURVIVAL MEDICINE

Handbook That Will Save Your Life In The Wilderness

Survival Medicine:
Handbook that will save your life in Wilderness

Introduction

Survival has always been a top priority for everyone. Whether you go for a camping in the forest or hiking or climbing in the back country, an essential survival skills and techniques play an important role. Even in case of a disaster or an epidemic, survival medicine comes very much in handy. For example, what would you do if you encounter any medical issue as a result of an epidemic or a calamity and you cannot see any ambulance or medical help coming your way? What if your family's health and well-being depends on you and your skills. Surely you won't sit back and just watch the sufferings in such situations. Here the survival medicine plays a major role. It can help you cope up with these circumstances and can save your life and that of your loved ones in situations where you are unable to find any medical doctor or help.

In recent years, human activities in wild have increased leading to a greater risk of illness and injuries. As a result, survival medicine has been developed considering both need and interest. This field is evolving day by day and is gaining a lot of attention and curiosity as more and more people are interested to know about it and want to learn different survival medicine skills and techniques. So, if you want to learn the ways by which you can save your life in wilderness than this book is the right choice as will guide you in understanding everything related to survival medicine in simple and easy language and in a better way.

Chapter 1 – What is Survival Medicine?

Researches in the field of science and medicine have led to the development of various drugs and antibiotics. Human life has been made better by the use of these medicines and mortality rate has also been reduced. This has been made possible due to the availability of hospital and medical facilities with in an arm's reach. However, saving a life could become a challenge if the ambulance is not coming in your direction. At that time, only survival medicine will save your life. In this chapter, we will see what actually survival medicine is and why medical training is necessary for you.

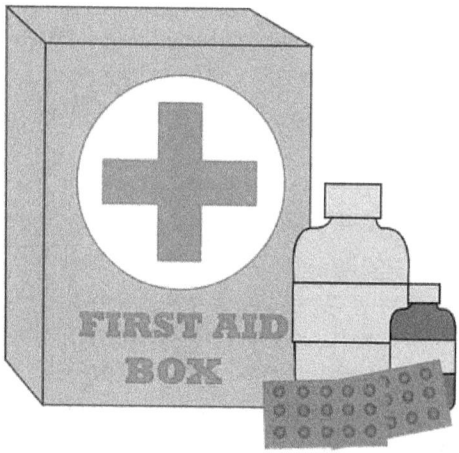

Survival medicine is the practice of medicine in remote settings and providing important emergency care when the professional medical support and facilities are miles away. The principle focus of this field is to evaluate, prioritize, treating serious injuries or illness and evacuating the victims in emergency.

Why survival medical training is important?

In order to understand any disease and injury, you should have enough knowledge of it. Therefore, medical training becomes necessary. The more you know, the more you would be in a better position to understand the situation you are in. You should have the information regarding the basic first aid. Moreover, the knowledge about the anatomy and physiology will be useful for you in acting more quickly and efficiently.

As a prudent medic for your group, you will take along with you a store of medication that will include both pharmaceutical and natural to use in serious settings. You should have antibiotics, pain relievers, anti-diarrheal and many other medicines with you. Furthermore to make the job easier, medical equipment, dressings, and agents for blood clotting etc. will very much come in handy. Along with it some dental equipment will also be essential. As far as medical preparedness is considered, these are some of the major steps.

The most important thing required to become a capable medic for your group is common sense. A sensible person having all the required supplies, knowledge and willingness to learn can become an efficient medical resource whenever his/her family is in crisis situation. As part of medical training, spend some time in emergency room. Learn CPR and how to take care of wounds and close them. Such a person who has emergency training and right supplies would be more useful than a doctor. It is necessary to mention here the important point to keep in mind regarding the survival medicine is to keep a calming deportment as the caregiver has to deal with agitated sick and injured people.

A useful characteristic of a good medic is his dedication to teach others some basic survival medicine skills. You cannot provide medical help to everyone at once so cross training also play a vital role here, as you may also be in need a medic one day.

Lastly, have faith in yourself and don't let anyone break it by saying that you won't become a successful medic in austere settings. If the professional are not available and you are the end of line when the wellbeing of your family and loved ones is at stake then be ready for that as you might be one who saves a life.

Chapter 2 – Major areas of Survival Medicine

Survival medicine is a vast field that is evolving day by day. It incorporates many areas of interests. Some of these focus on area like floods, landslides, storms, snow slip etc. while other focuses on broader areas like traumas. In this chapter, we will discuss some major areas of interest that comes under survival medicine. So here it goes.

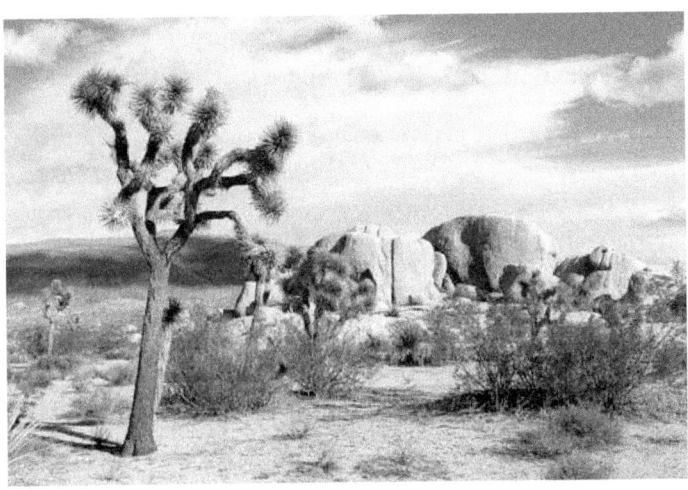

- **Increased height**

Traveling to high altitude is common and increasing day by day. As a result we see that the occurrence of acute mountain sickness is also high. High-altitude pulmonary edema (HAPE) and high-altitude cerebral edema (HACE) though are less common but are popular for being more serious conditions that can even be life threatening. These conditions are treated by moving downwards and administrating oxygen.

- **Diving**

Diving into sea and ocean is becoming popular worldwide for both refreshment and technical purposes. This may cause injuries like barotrauma and decompression illness. Barotrauma is the physical injury that is caused due to difference in air pressure and mostly affect ear and lungs whereas decompression illness refers to the condition that is caused due to reduction in ambient pressure surrounding the body. Inner ear decompression illness occurs more frequently. It is treated by recompressions in hyperbaric chamber.

- **Envenomation**

Envenomation refers to the process in which venom is injected into the body of a human or animal by the sting or bite of a venomous animal. There exist the variation in the detection and diagnosis of the marine envenomation, snake bites as well as arthropod stings and it depends on the way it is managed based on its location. The variation is due to the availability or lack of anti-venoms. These envenomation may cause coagulopathy or respiratory arrest and in more severe situation a cardiovascular collapse.

- **Trauma related Wilderness**

Wilderness can also cause trauma which may results from a head injury due to falling from a height during rock climbing, hiking or snow related activities. Mostly, the traumas are minor and less severe but they may stop outdoor activities as well as long trips. Sometimes they may become life threatening for example in case of prolonged harness suspension. Techniques such as shoulder reduction and many others are being taught to the caregivers as a part of survival medicine.

- **Hyperthermia**

Hyperthermia may also be related to wilderness. It is a condition in which the body temperature becomes elevated due to failed thermoregulation. In hyperthermia, more heat is absorbed or released by the body than it dissipates. Too much heat exposure can cause a number of illnesses like heat cramps, heat strokes etc. Some of these can be severe as well. To deal with these condition, removal from heat exposure and rapid cooling of whole body is used in which whole body is immersed in ice or cold water. However, such techniques are not possible in wilderness settings. So in these situations, patient's body temperature is lowered by extreme fanning and skin wetting.

- **Hypothermia**

Hypothermia is another worry in wilderness medicine. It refers to the condition which is caused due to extreme exposure to cold resulting in dangerous drop in body temperature. The fundamentals of hypothermia recovery comprise inhibition of further loss of heat and rewarming.

In some cases, prolonged recovery will be successful in obtaining a positive neurologic result. But, the required facilities are not available in wilderness settings.

- **Frostbite**

Frostbite is a complicated process that refers to body injuries caused due to exposure to extreme cold. It mostly affects nose, ear, fingers and toes. Basic care in wilderness settings includes the treatment of hypothermia along with the application of anti-prostaglandins, pain control and placing protective dressings.

- **Avalanche**

Avalanche refers to the fall or slide of a large mass of materials like snow, rock, ice or soil down the side of the mountain rapidly and suddenly. It is mostly common in mountainous terrain having thirty five percent slopes. Victims of avalanche become exposed to great traumatic forces leading to suffocation and hypothermia. Its severity depends on many factors like length of burial, depth of burial etc. Advancement has been made in the avalanche rescue and recovery due to improvements in understanding of snow burial physiology.

- **Battlefield medicine**

In the past decade, dramatic and radical advancement has been made in the battlefield medicine. It also includes the development of victim care guidelines and training. Major advances have been accomplished in hemorrhage control with bandages and hemostatic means, needle decompression, pain management, low-volume field recovery and in many others. Wilderness medicine is also making use of these advances.

- **Epidemiology**

Epidemiology plays an important role in wilderness settings and describes the prevalence of rate of death and disease. Work is still been done on collecting detailed information however general trends are available and can be described. Soft tissue lesions like blisters, strains, sprains and fractures are very common. Furthermore, head trauma, hyperthermia, hypothermia, cardiac arrest, suicide and drowning are the shared causes of death. This information comes very much in handy for general educational program, planning a trip, preparing a medical kit and reducing the severity of the risk.

- **Search and rescue operations**

Search and rescue operation in wilderness are conducted usually by volunteer groups. Member's medical training includes basic first aid, wilderness first aid, paramedic, mid-level provider etc. Search and rescue operations are mostly carried out for finding missing children, tourists as well as for individuals with psychological problems like autism, Alzheimer's disease or dementia. Search management has advanced a lot in recent years. Moreover, if possible, helicopters enable the prompt identification and rescue, provided they are positioned under proper circumstances.

- **Wilderness related travel medicine**

Travel medicine refers to the occurrence, distribution and control of traveler's diseases, education and application of vaccines. This field has gain popularity in the current period due to easy long distance travel. In travel medicine, malaria is principally important disease. It carries high rates of morbidity and mortality particularly in children.

- **Wilderness disaster medicine**

A substantial similarity exists between disaster medicine and wilderness medicine. Both play a major role in sudden, unpredicted, challenging and serious conditions. The outcomes of disaster result in number of diseases that are usual in wilderness settings or remote circumstances. Disaster management also involves the fundamentals of hygiene and cleanliness of water. These are also important along with many others.

- **Ultrasound**

Detailed examination of patients is carried out with the help of small, portable ultrasound machines. This technology is reported to be used extensively by US military in small remote receiving centers. Due to lack of resources, ultrasound has been used by disaster management in the remote settings.

Chapter 3 –Building a Survival medical kit

A survival medical kit is an important need for everyone as misfortune strikes without telling anyone. No matter where you are or what you are doing, if you are concerned about the survival then you will surely carry a survival medical kit along with you. In this chapter, we will tell you about how to build an effective medical kit for survival. Let's begin.

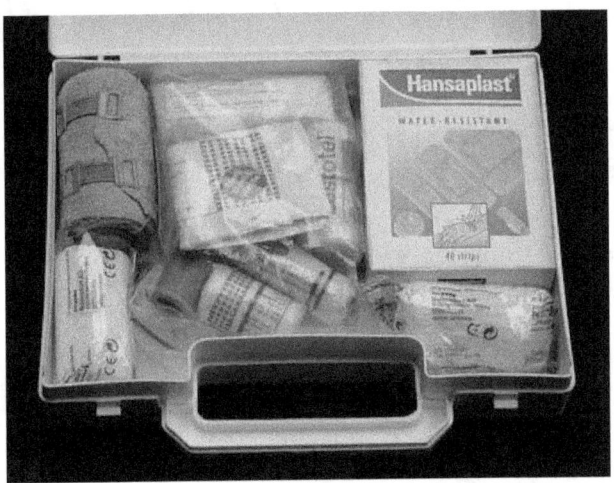

Medical knowledge can come in handy while building a medical kit for survival but not everybody has this skill. The important point is to know how to use the things that are inside the kit.

Essential Resources

The essentials resources are the ones that are mostly used. They cover a wide range of diseases like headaches, diarrhea, small cuts, inflammations etc. Owing to their excessive use, they should be place where they are easily available. Make it sure that you pack some extras as well. You can easily buy these supplies at any drugstore or pharmacy.

Medical equipment

While packing a medical kit, you must have these tools with you as they will come in handy in remote settings. These are thermometer, Q-tips, Stethoscope, tweezers, nail clippers, scalpel with blades, scissors and large trauma shears.

Important medications and lotions

While going on a journey, medicines and lotions play a very vital role in order to cope up with the diseases and causalities. This will be discussed in detail in the next chapter.

Wounds and Trauma

It is not easy to treat wounds or trauma as it requires a great level of medical training. Wounds can become unpleasant while traumas can be disturbing. However, in wilderness settings when the professional help is not available and it becomes your responsibility than do not panic. Following tools will help you out in these situations.

1) Treating blisters

For treating blisters, molefoam, moleskin, 2nd skin and medical tape play an important role.

2) Treating wounds

For treating wounds, Nitrile gloves, Triangle bandages, Sterile gauze pads, Medical tape, Israeli bandage, Band-Aids, Alcohol wipes, Ace Bandages, Tegaderm, Irrigation syringe, Steri-strip or butterfly closures, Sam-splint moldable foam splint, Suture kit, Iodine, Tourniquet are very vital and comes in handy.

Prescription Medicines

When building your survival medical kit, you must have some prescription medicines packed inside. Although you need some medical knowledge to administer these medications but if it will helpful in keeping them in medical kit as they will come in handy in the field. Some of these medicines include Epinephrine that are helpful in treating extreme allergic reactions, Ciprofloxacin and Azithromycin that are used for treating infections and Bactrim d.s. etc.

Personal Medicines

Personal medicines are of great importance where your own life is considered. These include asthma inhalers if you have breathing difficulties, multi-vitamins and epinephrine for allergic reactions.

Keeping a small toy or puzzle can help keep the children busy and calm them down in emergency situations as they can be a distraction. This can work just as good as any other medication. Occasionally, it can also be used with adults.

Toiletries such as toothpaste, tooth brush, razors and many others can also make a big difference in survival. Moreover, camp soap, lighter or waterproof matches, mosquito repellants, sun block etc. can also come in handy.

Maintaining your medical kit

Another important step while building your medical kit is storing all the things properly. Spend some time on thinking it properly and place everything in order and in a way that it is easily accessible to you.

Selecting a medical container

Selecting a right container that suits you the best according to your needs is very important step. Major factors to consider in this are size, shape, intention and weight. You want to select something that will be convenient for you to carry along in your trips. If you want a water proof medical kit then dry bags are great choice. Another durable and most functional container for medical kit is military medic bag pack. Choosing a medical container may appears to be an ordinary decision but it can protect you in survival settings.

Categorizing the medical kit

It is important to have an organized medical kit. In wilderness settings, time is very crucial. You cannot waste it by going through your unorganized kit to find your desired medicine or drug. Therefore, it is wise to categorize your kit into different groups like trauma, prescription medicine, personal medicine etc.

Furthermore, separating your categories can also help you solve many problems. You can do so by number of ways.

- **Using stuff sacks:** Stuff sacks are great for storage as they vary in their sizes and colors. They are extremely durable, light and most of them are water proof as well. They are also easily available in the market.
- **Using Tupperware:** If you are less concerned about the space and weight of your medical kit, then Tupperware will be a best choice for you.

They also vary in their sizes, shapes and colors. Moreover, they are also comparatively cheap and easily available.

- **Using zip lock bags:** They have many purposes. They are helpful in assembling and marking different drugs and bandages. They can be labeled with the help of a marker. Additionally, they are best for keeping the liquid medicine or drug's bottles that can leak.
- **Using Pill bottles:** These bottles are excellent for keeping the medicines. They are inexpensive as well as economical and reusable. Bands aids and other small objects can easily be arranged by the usage of these bottles.

Updating your medical kit

Your work does not end just after building a medical kit that can save your life in wilderness and emergency situations. Every medicine and drug has an expiration date. Medicines that have expired will be of no help to you in emergency satiations especially in remote settings. Sometimes, the seal of the container may fail and cause a leakage that can ruin your supplies. It is best to keep your medical kit up to date and replacing whatever is needed by checking out the expiry dates of medicines and container seals. An easy way to do it is by making a checklist. This will be helpful in keeping the track of the medicines that you have or that you need and what the expiry dates of certain medicines are.

Purchasing a Pre-packed survival medical kit

Buying a pre-made survival kit can be very helpful and efficient and can save you from a lot of hassle. Today, many high quality and relatively affordable medical kits like North American Rescue CCRK, Dixiegear First Responder Trauma Kit etc. are available in the market for use in survival settings. You can customize them according to your needs and requirements by adding extras.

In short, whether you buy a pre-made medical kit or build your own, it will cost you some money but it will be worth spending considering when your life is at stake in wilderness settings.

Chapter 4 – Essential medications for your Survival medical kit

Misfortune strikes without telling. Before you know it you may be in an emergency situation in remote settings. It is always wise to prepare yourself well in order to handle these situations. This also involves carrying with you an emergency kit that has the entire essential over the counter (OTC) medicines for emergency situations.

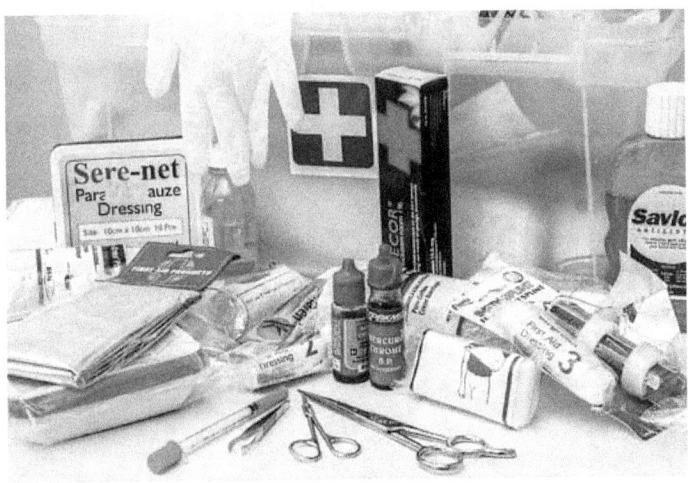

In this chapter, we will discuss all the OTC medications that will come in handy to save your life in wilderness survival conditions.

1) Aspirin

Aspirin or acetylsalicylic acid (ASA) is a common medicine. It is a cheap non-prescription medication in history. It helps in reducing fever, pain and in treating inflammation. In case of fever or pain, it begins to effect within thirty minutes. It lowers the risk of cancers like colorectal cancer. It is excellent for thinning of blood. It helps in recovering from a heart attack and also inhibits the risk of future attacks and strokes. Due to these benefits, you should have both adult and children aspirin in your medical kit.

2) Ibuprofen

Another best OTC medicine for your survival kit is Ibuprofen. It works to lower the pain, fever and inflammation. It is also used in treating painful menstrual cramps, migraine and rheumatoid arthritis. It affects usually starts within an hour.

3) Antacids

In wilderness settings it is not surprising that you may get gassy tummies or stomach acidity. This may be caused due to stress and lack of food. Antacids can help you with stomach acidity and indigestion. It can also help you get relieve from heartburns. This over the counter medicine is usually taken by mouth.

4) Antihistamines and anti-allergens

Allergies become very common in wilderness remote settings. You cannot stop it from happening but can control it. Antihistamines are great for getting rid of them. They are helpful in treating allergic reactions to nose like itching, running nose etc. They are also used to treat insomnia and gastric acid conditions.

5) Bismuth Subsalicylate

Bismuth subsalicylate is also known as Pink bismuth. It helps in treating many digestive system issues. This includes the treatment of diarrhea, ingestion, heartburns and nausea. Today it is also available in the form of a pill that is more convenient to carry with you.

6) Cough and mucus control

Cough and mucus control medicine comes in the form of both pills and syrups. This medicine can save you from visiting a doctor as well as from the bill. It may result due to different allergies, influenza, sinus infections and exposure to many other conditions. It provides relief to a person who is suffering and also protect the others who are healthy as the disease has better chances of spread via coughing.

7) Laxatives

Laxatives are very important over the counter medicines that help in relieving your discomfort. In wilderness settings, constipation can occur due to different kinds of food intake. Constipation can be threatening if it is not treated. Laxatives are usually taken by mouth and helps in treating and preventing constipation.

8) Sleep aids

Insomnia and many other sleep related disorders may result in disaster and wilderness settings. Its main reason is the stress caused due to surroundings conditions. It becomes difficult for you to fall sleep and stop thinking about the survival situations you are in. Lack of sleep may affect your ability to think and make good decisions and judgments. So sleep becomes even more important. There are many sleeping pills that can help you with the sleeping issues. Make it sure you choose the one that is best for you. It is also best for you to keep natural remedies like lavender oil etc. in your survival kit.

9) Saline solutions

Saline solution is a mixture of salt and water. It has various medical benefits. It is considered as an important OTC medicine to keep in your bag. It helps in washing the wounds and eye and sinus flushing. It is also used to remove the contact lenses.

10) Vitamins

Vitamins are the most important over the counter medicine to have with you in survival settings. Organic vitamins are taken to control the vitamin deficiency in body that results in post-disaster scenario. Therefore, it is important that you carry your favorite multi-vitamins with you in your medical kit.

All the above medicines can easily be bought from the market and do not require any prescription. Make it sure that your medical kit is updated and contains the medicines that are not expired. You surely do not want to carry the expired burden of medicines that would be of no help to you in survival conditions. Lastly, do keep extras in your medical kit in case someone comes to you for help in emergency situations.

Chapter 5 – Skills required for Survival Medicine

This chapter will talk about the basic skills that are required for survival medicine. They can help you in coping up with the emergency situations that may occur in remote setting. Nobody wants to get stuck in misfortune but it is better to be prepared ahead of time in order to tackle these unwanted circumstances that you might face in wilderness settings.

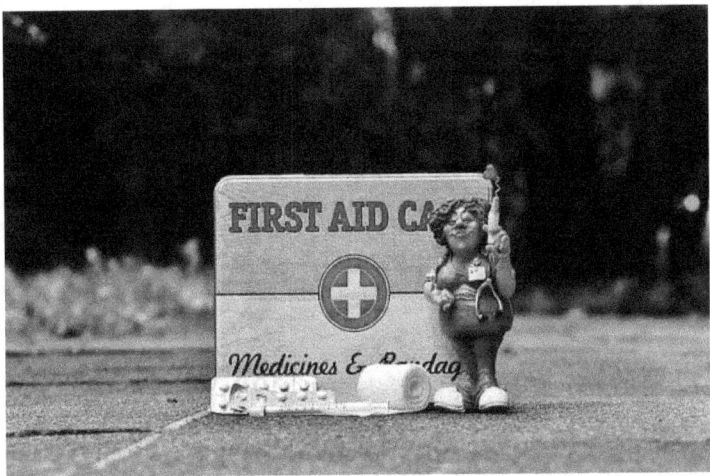

Strong will power

The first and the foremost important skill in survival medicine is the strong will to survive. Maintaining a calm state of mind is very essential factor for survival. In addition, a common factor that we see in all the remarkable survival stories is the strong survival will power. Optimism and positive attitude will help you in better thinking. As a result of it, you will be able to make good decisions and right judgments and would be in a better position to survive.

Basic needs

Fulfilling the basic needs is another important skill for survival. In wilderness survival, there are four basic needs. These are food, warmth, water and sleep.

- **Food:**
  Food is very important for survival. It provides energy to your body and helps you to fight with the surrounding misfortunes. Although human body can go without food for days but it will make your body weak and will affect your ability to think.
- **Warmth:**
  Maintaining your body temperature is also an important skill for survival. In most of the wilderness settings, it becomes a challenge to keep your body warm particularly at night.
- **Water:**
  Water serves to be an important need for every human being. Although you can go without water for two to three days but it is wise to keep your water supply filled at all the times.
- **Sleep:**
  Sleep is also an important requirement of human beings for them to think rational and logical. Without a proper sleep you won't be able to make good decisions.

Overcoming Stress

Stress and tension are very common in wilderness disaster settings. The basic rule for survival is to overcome this stress before it start impacting your mind and decision making.

Building a shelter

Whenever you face a survival situation then the first priority is to build the shelter. A good shelter will protect you from a number of factors like weather conditions, animals and insects etc. Furthermore, it should be comfortable for sleeping and resting.

Making a fire

An important skill to learn is how to make fire. Making fire can help resolve many problems for you like keeping the animals and insects away from you. It can help you in cooking the food and purifying the water. You can also sterilize your bandages with its help.

Finding water

As mentioned before that water is very important for human beings. Finding water before your supply finishes is another skill for survival. Without it, you may likely suffer from dehydration that can even become life threatening. There are many indicators for finding the water for example birds, insects, green vegetation, muddy ground etc.

Finding food in the wild

In the wilderness settings you must have some skills for finding food as it is necessary for your mental state and provide you energy. Take benefit of everything that is edible around you like plants, insects, meat etc. but be careful regarding the poisonous plants that can be harmful for you.

Signaling for help

For any survival situation, you must learn and practice the skill of signaling for help. There are countless ways by which you can signal for help whenever in emergency situation. You can either use fire, smoke, signal lights or flashlights to signal for your rescue.

Basic first aid

In emergency situations, you must have knowledge about using basic first aid even if you are stressed. Information regarding how to treat small injuries and wounds can make a huge difference. Furthermore, controlling the severe causalities can help a lot as well.

Knowing the weather

Predicting the weather can help you dealing with the survival situations. Avoiding the bad weather can save you from many troubles and problems.

Navigation

Another important skill to learn is finding your way in the wilderness by using the surrounding factors. You can find your directions by using sun, moon, stars, trees, wind and many others. This skill can come very much in handy in wilderness.

Managing your fear

Managing your fear is another important skill in wilderness. The emergency situations inculcate fear and panic in human beings. Only by managing your fear you can move ahead and think more rational and logical.

Wilderness survival training

Just knowing the skills is not enough for you to deal with survival situations. You must practice them as well. By joining different courses that are taught in wilderness survival school can help you to prepare for any disastrous situations.

Conclusion

Hence, we can say that survival medicine play an important role in our lives. Human beings only have one life. You cannot waste it by just giving up or not doing anything. Life is a struggle but whoever is able to survive these challenges become the real heroes. You cannot avoid what is bound to happen nor can you know about it ahead of time. The only thing you can do is to prepare yourself for the worst scenarios and situations. When you are already prepared to deal with the worst situations only then you can enjoy your life to its fullest with fewer worries.

This book will provide you a guidance that can save your life in the wilderness settings. It will tell you the knowledge regarding what is survival medicine and why it is necessary. You will also get to know about some areas of survival medicine. It will also guide you in building a proper medical kit that is best for survival in remote settings. The information related to essential over the counter medication is also packed in this book. Lastly, it will also tell you about different skills that are important for survival.

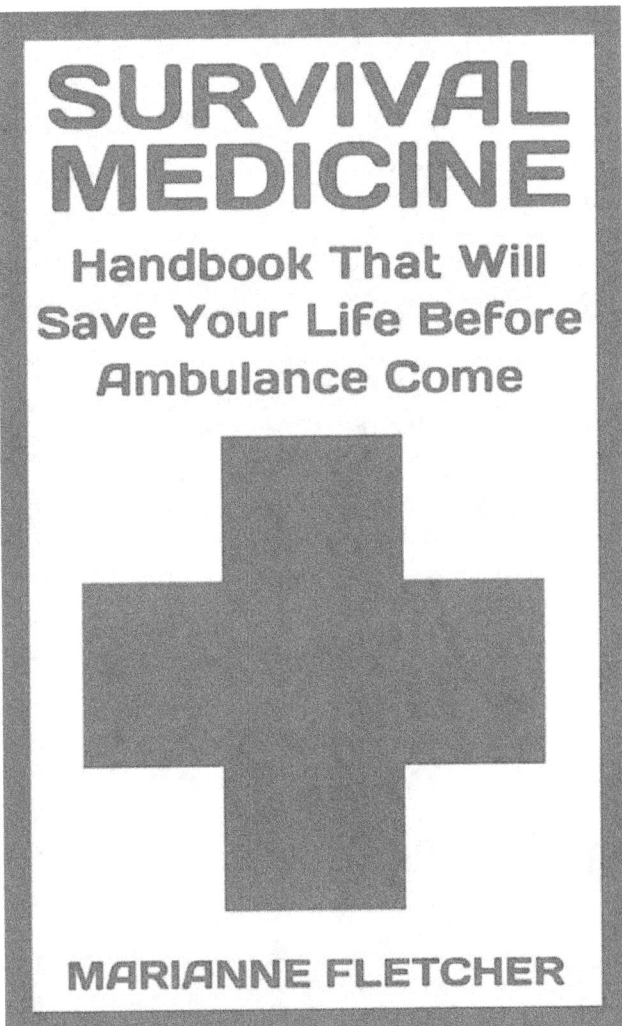

Survival Medicine:

Handbook That Will Save Your Life Before Ambulance Come!

Introduction

I would like to thank and congratulate you on downloading *"Survival Medicine: Handbook that Will Save Your Life Before Ambulance Come!"* This book is a great handbook that offers you all kinds of tips and suggestions on how you can prepare survival medicine in an emergency. Gaining this knowledge and skills will certainly be most beneficial if you find yourself in a wilderness where you have perhaps lost contact with civilization and must rely on your own first aid skills to survive this ordeal you may find yourself in.

You just never know when you could find yourself in a situation where you need to do some basic first aid on yourself or others while waiting for an ambulance to arrive or medical help of some sort. It is very important when you are going outside of the protection of civilization to explore the wilderness. During times like this it is vital that you and your group have prepared by making sure to bring a first aid kit on your adventure. I am sure you will find the tips and suggestions within these pages most helpful to you in helping to guide you on how to prepare emergency survival medicine and treatments.

Chapter 1. Building Your Basic First Aid Kit

If you find yourself in a medical emergency when in the wilderness, it is vital that you are prepared to help ensure that you will have the best tolls available. You can build your own first aid kit or you can purchase a prepared kit. You should make sure that your first aid kit has the following items included in it:

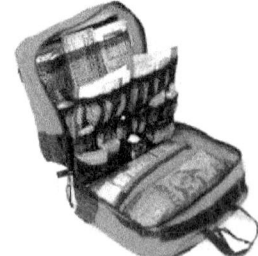

- Latex gloves, have lots of pairs as you do not want to re-use them.
- Roll of 1-inch wide athletic tape. Bring about 1 roll per person. It works great for dressing wounds, prevents blisters, and will help to support joints such as twisted ankle.
- Rolled gauze to maintain a dressing for wounds.
- Sterile wrapped gauze pads in variety of sizes. Make sure to have some that are non-adherent, as they are suitable for certain types of wounds.
- Scissors
- Tweezers
- A tourniquet
- Over the counter meds such as topical antibiotic cream, gastrointestinal medications, anti-diarrheal, pain relievers, antihistamines, and stomach soothing medications. Pack your kit in a waterproof container.

Wound Care

When faced with a wound in the wilderness, there are two initial priorities: controlling the bleeding, and preventing infection. Bleeding must be controlled quickly to help minimize the chance of the injured person going into shock or dying from blood loss. Infection must be prevented from setting into the wound, so that bacteria will not multiply and make the injured party sick.

Control Bleeding

If there is a wound that is bleeding freely take a gauze and apply pressure to the wound with it. If possible try to elevate the wound above the height of the individual's heart, this will help to slow the blood flow. If the pressure is not stopping the bleeding, you may need to apply a tourniquet. Using a tourniquet should only be used as a last resort. The use of tourniquets can result in the need for an amputation or other complications. However, if the risk of death due to blood loss is a threat, and other methods are not working a tourniquet is necessary.

Infection Prevention

Once you have managed to control the bleeding, it is very important to take proactive steps to make sure that infection is prevented. These steps include cleaning the wound with soap and water, rinsing it clear of any foreign objects, using tweezers if needed. Keep irrigating the wound with water, and rinsing it with iodine.

Treating Shock

A person will go into medical shock due to loss of blood or insufficient blood flow throughout their body as well as other severe physiological stress. Blood loss, trauma, dehydration, head injury, and severe infections are just a few of the many situations which lead to a person going into shock.

Diagnosing Shock

You can tell if a person has gone into shock based on the following typical symptoms:

- Skin is pale
- Dizziness, disorientation, agitation
- Excessive thirst
- Hyperventilation
- Fainting

Treatment

If you believe that someone is going into shock, it is vital that you treat them. Shock can be life threatening if not treated. Below are some basic steps for treatment of shock:

1. Place the person suffering from shock onto their back. Elevate their legs six to eight inches above the level of their heart. If the person is unconscious, make sure to place them on their side or lying on their stomach with their head turned to the side. This is to help ensure that they will not choke on vomit or other fluids.

2. Any wet clothing the person is wearing remove it, and ensure they are comfortable. If it is cold weather, use blankets and other heat sources to warm the injured person. If it is hot out, try and find a shady spot for the person.

3. If the person is conscious keep them hydrated by giving them fluids, preferably containing salt or sugar.

4. Allow the person to get some rest until they recover.

When to Evacuate

If you do experience injury or illness while in the wilderness, it is a good idea to add an evacuation plan or have one in place. Make sure that you tell friends and family where you are going to be or location. This is important because you may not be able to contact them in an emergency so they need to know where to begin searching for you. If you do get contact, ask what is the best way for you to approach medical treatment.

Chapter 2. First Aid Vs. Survival Medicine

There is a difference between caring for an injured person after an earthquake, until the first responders arrive to caring for that person from the start of them becoming injured or sick right through until they make their recovery. There are many first aid courses offered for the public to take. In the US, most volunteer ambulance departments are constantly looking for new recruits. The Red Cross teaches first aid, in many countries, often with a focus on disasters.

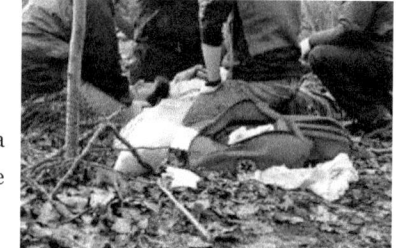

If you want to give your first aid knowledge a good boost, seeking out such a course would be a great idea.

First Aid

First aid is the immediate response to an emergency or sudden illness. It helps to save the patient, ensuring that they will be given the best treatment to help ensure that they will survive the ordeal they are in.

First aid is a very essential skill, it is your immediate response to a serious medical problem. You will need to diagnose the problem, and remove any immediate dangers that could cause further damage or even death to the victim.

If you find yourself in the middle of an emergency, you will follow the strategy known to first responders: stabilize the patient and ready them for transportation. You will prepare the victim to be transported to a medical facility where they will be able to get more in depth treatment.

Outback Medicine

Not all disasters happen within a civilized region. You could be involved in a plane crash, where you are asked to help provide aid for other passengers. If you are stranded somewhere far from civilization, you might become the only hope that the injured person has for surviving. You will need to factor in the follow-up care to keep the injured party stable until help does arrive.

Survival Medicine

The third scenario is where it is assumed that help is not coming. This would be a safe assumption in a situation where you are in the middle of a large-scale disaster that has cut you off from civilization or you are one of very few survivors. In this scenario, you are needed at the site of the initial injury. Not only are you going to have to stabilize the injury, but you will need to continue your care until the injured party is cured or controlled.

You will need to know how to tackle chronic conditions such as thyroid and arthritis problems, heart disease and chicken pox. Survival medicine is an all-encompassing skill with a different approach to basic first aid.

First Aid Strategy

When you are a first responder to an accident, illness, or injury, there is a basic order of duties that you must follow. As the first responder, you are the primary caregiver, whether it is a full collapse of civilization or a car crash, it is your job to see that you and your patient emerge in the best condition possible given the circumstances that you are in.

It is important that you and your patient's safety is important, so the set of principles that you follow will be your mantra. When you find, yourself faced with a need to employ your first aid skills, whether it is until help arrives or for the long term, the following are steps you must follow:

1. **Assess the situation.** Study the scene you are faced with, be on the look-out for any dangers or hazards that could put you or your patient at risk. For example, make sure that you will not be hit by falling debris while you are trying to reach your patient.

2. **Remove immediate dangers.** To help ensure that the situation does not become even worse, make sure to remove any immediate dangers before you begin to administer treatment. Remember that your own safety is just as important as your patient's safety. If you too, become injured their chances of survival are greatly reduced or lost all together. Put out fires, and remove debris, move your patient to a safer location if you cannot secure the scene itself.

3. **Protect yourself from becoming contaminated.** Since you do not know fully what you are dealing with, protect yourself before you administer aid. Using a mask, gloves and apron are very important medical tools, not only will they help to prevent contaminated fluids from contacting you, but they will also protect your patient from becoming contaminated from your body.

4. Assess for life threatening injuries. What you need to assess right away if there is anything that could be threatening your patient's life. There is no use spending time diagnosing a compound fracture, for example, if your patient in the meantime is bleeding out due to a severed artery. You will need to check the following:

Airway—is there anything that could be preventing your patient from inhaling oxygen? Check to make sure that there are no objects in their mouth or throat that are blocking their airway.

Breathing—check to make sure that your patient is breathing normally.

Circulation—is your patient breathing normally? Check to see if there is any severe bleeding that could be life threatening to your patient.

Extreme injury—check to see if your patient has a neck or head injury that needs to be stabilized to help ensure their survival.

Exposure—is your patient exposed to an environmental or any external threat that could be life threatening?

5. Treat life threatening issues. You must immediately deal with any life-threatening issues, before you continue with your diagnosis and first aid. Before you begin a deeper examination of your patient, it is vital that you get them stabilized first.

6. Perform a thorough examination of situation. The injured person may not be able to communicate to you their injuries, because they might be unconscious. If they are conscious ask them what happened, and where they are hurt. This will offer you some help in diagnosing the situation, but keep in mind that your patient may not be aware of all their injuries. Some injuries can cause paralysis or numbness. When you examine the patient's body more thoroughly it will help you to become aware of the less obvious injuries.

7. Administer aid. Perform first aid on your patient's injuries, as well as treating them for things such as shock and hypothermia. Your goal here is to stabilize the patient and give them the best chance for recovery. Except in extreme conditions, the patient's long term care will take place in another location.

8. Make plans to evacuate. If help is on the way you will not have to worry about transporting your patient. However, if you need to transport them to a safe location, you need to plan to do this in such a way to prevent any part of the patient's injuries worsening in the process.

9. Transport the patient. First you need to make sure that your patient is stable and secure before you attempt to move them. This is especially true when you are dealing with a neck or back injury, moving the person could cause severe damage. You might have to create a shelter where you are so that you can treat the patient in place. If you feel that the patient is stable enough to move, make sure that any broken limbs are secured, and bandages will stay in place.

Chapter 3. The Principles of First Response

While you are following, the guidelines covered in the previous chapter to successfully treat your patient at the scene of the accident or their injury, you need to follow a set of principles. These principles will help you to improve your chances of success— and can leave your patient in the best condition possible. Here is a guideline of principles to try and follow:

- **Remain calm.** It is not always easy to remain calm, but it is imperative. By remaining calm you will make better decisions, and will be aware of more details and will certainly be more productive when you are in a calm state of mind. When we hurry and rush through things we often make more mistakes. We also must keep in mind what your reaction will have on the patient. The last thing you want to do is cause the patient to become even more panicked than they are ready are. It could cause them to move and in the process, could add to their injuries and also have a negative effect on their heart rate.

- **Involve the patient.** Keeping your patient involved is important, because they are more aware of what happened to them than you are. Their help can be invaluable when it comes to you treating their injuries. The patient can also inform you of hidden issues, for example, a blood clotting disease that could increase the time it will take for the wound to heal. They can inform you if they have a headache or they feel nauseated, you cannot see these, but they can help you in your diagnosis. When you involve the patient, it can help to keep them calm and quell their fears. It is a show of respect to ask the patient's permission before you begin treatment and to explain your progress as you go. Keep in mind that it is not your body and you have no right to touch it. It is best, if possible to seek the permission to do so from the patient first.

- **Seek information.** Even if your patient is unable to communicate with you, there are still clues you can search for. Assess the scene, try to figure out what led to these injuries, and why?

  It can often help you to give a better diagnosis or even allow you to spot more subtle injuries to the patient. Check the patient for medical cards or bracelets that may alert you to pre-existing medical conditions.

- **Assume the worst.** Pessimism in a first aid situation is certainly useful. It is a good idea to assume that the patient has serious injuries such as a broken neck or back. Better that you go the extra mile to move a patient onto a stretcher than to discover too late, as you help them to stand, that a neck injury was present all along.

- **Enlist help.** Speed can certainly be an important criterion, especially if you are in a crisis, and you need to get the patient to a safe location as quickly as possible. Other people may not be medically trained, but they still can assist you with many of the tasks you may need to perform. It is seldom a good idea to move a patient on your own, unless you have no choice.

- **Take charge.** If you are enlisting help, make sure that you establish yourself as being the medical authority in the situation. Explain to others that you are taking charge of the situation, as a first responder and have the situation under control. Use an authoritative tone, and request assistance from others, explaining what you need and why. You can relinquish your authority if you discover that there are more qualified medical professionals within the group. It is never a bad idea to defer to greater knowledge and experience.

- **Consider all dangers.** Accidents rarely happen in safe areas. Falls, crashes, and even disasters—these things have potential to harm you or anyone else on the scene. Never put yourself in harm's way or anyone else without good reason. For example, throwing yourself into a river filled with rapids is not going to save the victim. Always be on the alert for dangers, while treating the patient, move everyone to a safe location.

- **Think hard before moving the patient.** Before you consider moving from the scene, make sure that the patient is recovered enough to be moved. Injuries could become more serious if a patient is moved. One of the most difficult choices you may have to make is deciding whether to move your patient. You need to gather as much information as you can before you even consider moving them.

Chapter 4. First Aid & Medical Supplies

If you are the person that is responsible for first aid within your group, you will be responsible for making sure that your kit bag is equipped to administer care. You need to have enough supplies to last for the time where you will be unable to receive help from a medical facility.

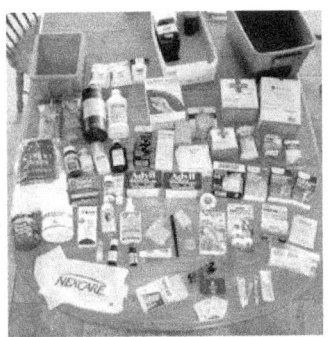

If you are heading out on an excursion with a group, you need to make sure that you have enough medical supplies to last a few days, before help can arrive. If you are stocking a shelter that you are planning to use as a residence after a disaster or collapse, you will need to stock it up with months, if not years of supplies.

For those everyday maladies and small aches and pains, you will need:

- Aspirin for aches and pains and heart problems
- Painkillers (also have a child friendly version if you have young children)
- Benadryl for allergic reactions
- Flu and severe cold remedies
- Diarrhea medicine
- Adrenaline injectors
- Antibiotics
- Women's feminine hygiene products
- Diapers for baby and other care products for infants

- Stomach upset remedy
- Good quality skin lotion
- Calamine lotion
- Burn gel or spray
- Aloe Vera gel for sunburn
- Potassium iodide tablets
- Silver sulfadiazine cream
- Soap and hand sanitizer
- Celox combat gauze
- Topical antifungal powder or ointment
- Steroid cream
- Antihistamines
- A supply of any medications that you or others in your family or party, take regularly such as insulin or heart medication.

For treatment of wounds and other emergencies:

- Plenty of bandages, they will need to be changed regularly
- Band Aids and dressings
- Hemostatic products for serious bleeds
- A hemostat clamp
- Scalpels and a field knife
- Splints and wraps for all limbs in case of breakages and sprains
- Towels
- Disinfectant, such as rubbing alcohol to clean wounds
- Medical tape
- Medical grade glue
- Eye pads
- A neck clamp
- A neck collar

- An epinephrine auto injector for severe allergic reaction
- Anticoagulant
- Activated charcoal
- Asthma inhaler
- A nylon suture
- Corticosteroid tablets

General equipment for your medical room:

- A small flashlight
- Scissors
- Tweezers
- Sterilizing wipes for cleaning wounds
- A tourniquet
- Syringes and injection needles
- Scalpels and scalpel blades of various sizes
- A surgical mask for use during first aid and surgery
- A stethoscope
- A thermometer—one oral and one rectal
- Pen light or head lamp
- A stretcher
- Crutches
- Cold and hot compresses for swelling
- A thermal blanket for treating hypothermia
- Compression wraps
- A blood pressure cuff
- A glucose meter
- Cotton balls
- Petroleum jelly
- Safety pins

- Medical needle and thread for stitching wounds

Many of these items you can purchase in pharmacies and supermarkets or online. After a disaster locate the nearest medical supply center near your location. It is never recommended to administer such treatments under normal circumstances without having proper medical training, but when in a disaster scenario this calls for different behavior.

Chapter 5. Checking for Immediate Signals & Vital Signs

When you first encounter a patient, do not assume that you are seeing the full extent of their injuries. The patient may not complain of nothing more than a sprained ankle, but that does not mean you are safe to assume that there is nothing else wrong with the patient. We have all heard of internal bleeding stories, that have gone unnoticed until it was too late or the broken ankle that was walked on for two days before anyone realized it was more than just a sprained ankle.

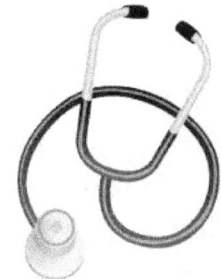

As a first responder, you need to assess the patient's full body, from head to toe. You need to assume the worst—an injury is guilty until it the first responder has proven it innocent. Checking your patient's vital signs is going to be your primary indicator of your patient's status. Checking to see if your patient's breathing, heart beat and blood pressure are all good. When you are starting your assessment of your patient these are the details you are going to want to stay focused on.

The vital signs of your patient will vary according to their age. In general, look for vital signs within the following ranges:

- Expect 30 to 50 breaths per minute from a newborn baby, a pulse between 120 to 160 beats per minute and blood pressure of 60 to 80.
- Expect 30 to 40 breaths per minute from a baby aged six months to a year, a pulse between 110 to 140 beats per minute, and blood pressure of 70 to 80.

- Expect 20 to 30 breaths from a toddler aged two to four, a pulse between 100 and 110 beats per minute, and blood pressure of 80 to 95.
- Expect 14 to 20 breaths per minute from a child between five and eight years old, a pulse between 90 and 100 beats per minute, and blood pressure of 90 to 100.
- Expect 12 to 20 breaths per minute from a child between the ages of eight and twelve years old, a pulse between 80 and 100 per minute, and blood pressure of 100 to 110.
- Expect 12 to 20 breaths per minute from a teenager between the ages of 12 to 18, with a pulse between 60 to 90 beats per minute, and blood pressure of 100 to 120.
- Expect 12 to 18 breaths per minute from an adult, with a pulse between 55 to 90 beats per minute, and blood pressure of 120.

You need to check off all the likely indicators of a problem when you first examine your patient. As a general rule try to follow these steps while you investigate the status of your patient's health:

1. Check for breathing: If your patient is unconscious, place your ear near to the nose and mouth to see if you can hear breath coming in and out. Watch their chest at the same time. Count the breaths according to your patient's vital signs. If the patient is not breathing or is struggling for breath, you will need to open the airway or breathe on their behalf. It is vital to steady the breathing as your patient will not be able to go without oxygen. If you hear strange sounds, such as rattling, there could be an obstruction in the throat that you will need to remove.

2. Check your patient's pulse. Using the tip of your middle finger and index fingers check for a pulse on the artery at the patient's wrist. If you are unable to locate one, check the inside of the upper arm (brachial artery), groin (femoral artery), or neck (carotid artery). If you cannot locate a pulse you will need to begin chest compressions immediately.

3. Look for bleeding. You should always check the heartbeat and breathing first with an unconscious patient. A conscious patient clearly has these functions to at least be good enough to be capable of speech. When you are dealing with a conscious patient, it is vital that you begin a dialogue with them immediately to help reassure them that they will be taken care of, and assure them of your intentions. Keep and eye out for any bleeding. Any sign of bleeding can be harmful, but it can be deadly if it is uncontrolled heavy bleeding. Examine the body of your patient to identify any areas that might be bleeding. These areas must be addressed as soon as possible.

4. Perform a full body evaluation of your patient. Move clothing around as much as you can without exposing the patient. Check for abnormalities on your patient's body, these could indicate fractures, wounds or other issues.

5. Check your patient's mental status. If your patient is awake, ask them questions to find out how lucid they are, such as their name, profession, and date. Listen to your patient's speech: if there is an abnormality such as slurring, this could be a symptom of a problem such as hypothermia.

6. Check your patient's blood pressure. When a person is at rest their average blood pressure should be 140/190. If it is too low this could indicate that your patient is in shock or is hemorrhaging.

7. Feel your patient's neck. Carefully and gently check your patient's vertebra and look for tenderness and muscles in spasm. Check their Adam's apple for a sensation almost like crunching. If you suspect that your patient has suffered a neck injury, immobilize the neck as quickly as possible. Sudden movements could exacerbate the problem and pain could cause your patient to twitch or try to move.

8. Check your patient's spine. Run your fingers down your patient's spine to check for back injuries. Press gently as you go down the spine, checking for tender areas. Ask your patient to move their limbs, and ask them if they have lost feeling in any areas. You can lightly pinch fingers and toes to see if your patient still has sensation. If there is loss of feeling this could indicate a back injury. This will require your patient to be immobilized as securely as possible—and kept in one position.

9. Check your patient for head injuries. Check the skull by pressing lightly around it to look for any areas on the skull or skin that are raised or depressed or are bleeding. Shine a light into your patient's eyes to make sure that both pupils are the same size and are responding to the light by constricting. If the pupils are small in your patient this could be a sign of an overdose or a brain injury. Pupils that are uneven can mean that the eye itself is injured or that your patient has a head injury. Check for other injuries on the head such as broken teeth, nose or swollen tongue.

10. Examine your patient's skin. Check for indicators such as abnormal skin color, bruises, bites, rashes or burns. Feel the temperature of your patient to check for fever. Press down on fingernails to check for circulation, pressing down will cause the skin to go white; if the circulation is normal, color will return to skin in two seconds.

If you pinch the skin and it remains loose, this could be an indication that your patient is dehydrated. Check inside of your patient's eyelids for a pale color that can indicate that there is internal bleeding or anemia.

11. Check your patient's chest. Check the chest area for any deformities, also observe the expanding and contracting of each breath that your patient takes.

12. Examine your patient's abdomen. Check for cuts and wounds, also press to see if there is any tenderness.

13. Check your patient's limbs and joints. Check each limb by pressing to check for tenderness, as well as the chest, ribs and collarbone.

14. Check your patient's temperature. By checking your patient's temperature this can indicate to you that not all is well with the patient's body. If your patient's temperature is too low this could indicate that they are suffering from hypothermia, while too high could mean hyperthermia or fever.

Whether you need to keep your patient from moving or not, it is best to assume that the situation will deteriorate with time. Repeat your examinations regularly, looking for new signs and signals, check to see if the symptoms that you are treating are not worsening or spreading.

Keep checking the mental status of your patient to make sure that they remain lucid. Do not leave your patient alone, if you need to get more supplies, ask someone to sit with your patient while you are gone.

Taking a first aid course is something that you will certainly not regret, as you will be taught how to treat injured people for many kinds of injuries, wounds, and other medical conditions. You will be instructed by medical professionals on how to perform such first aid treatments as CPR, Mouth to Mouth Resuscitation, Treat Shock, Recovery Position and much more first aid skills. These are certainly great skills to have especially when we live in such a world of uncertainty, we just don't know when and where the next disaster will strike. It will certainly feel good to know that you have prepared yourself for the worst, it is better to be safe than sorry. Learning these first responder skills will make you feel more secure knowing that you will be able to help those in need during an emergency.

Conclusion

I hope that you will find the tips and suggestions, on how to prepare for becoming a good first responder in an emergency useful to you in your time of need. I am sure that you will be happy that you learned these first aid skills and made the effort to be prepared for an emergency. You will gain much comfort in knowing that you are armed with the proper medical supplies and knowledge to be able to help others in need of your assistance in an emergency. A good start for preparing yourself would be to start by putting together your own emergency first aid kit.

I would like to thank you once again for downloading my book, your support of my work means a great deal to me. I would love to read a review of my book by you on Amazon. Take care and a I wish you great success in you developing your first responder skills.

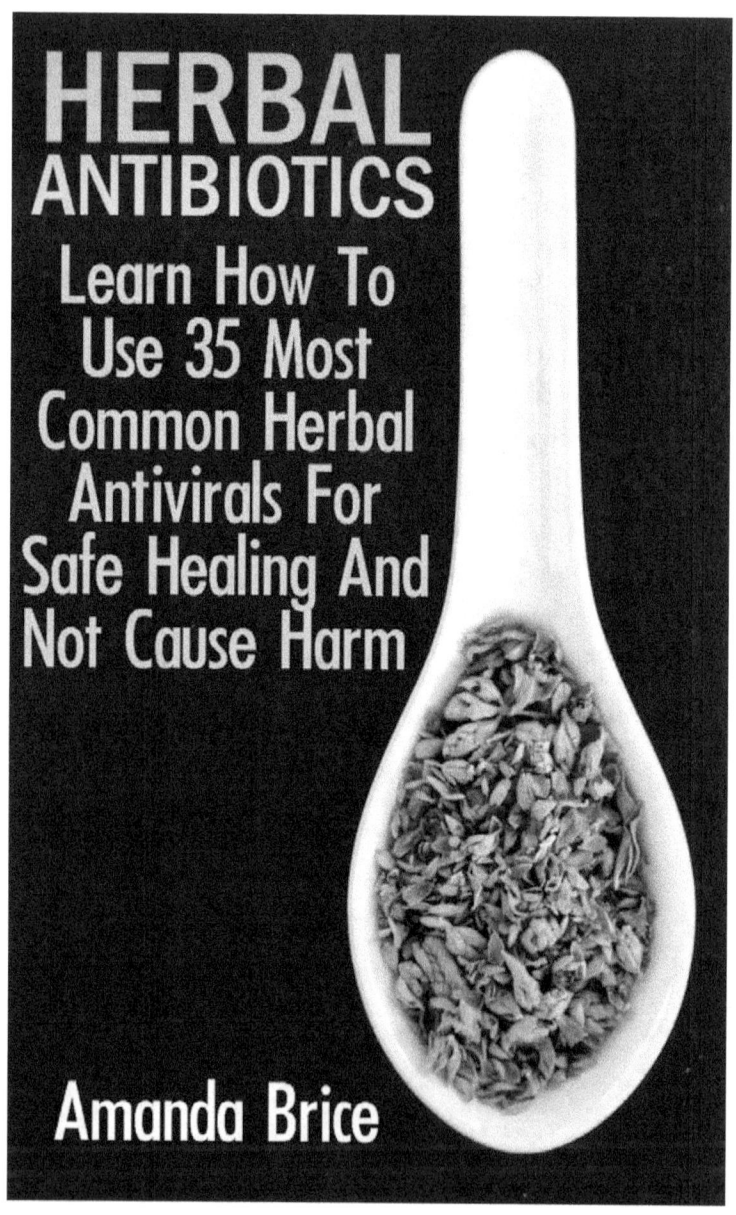

HERBAL
ANTIBIOTICS
Learn How To
Use 35 Most
Common Herbal
Antivirals For
Safe Healing And
Not Cause Harm

Amanda Brice

Herbal Antibiotics

Learn How To Use 35 Most Common Herbal
Antivirals For Safe Healing And Not To
Cause Harm

Introduction

You feel that little tickle in the back of your throat, and you sigh. You don't have time to get sick right now, and you certainly don't have time to feel groggy from your cold medicine. You have a life to live, and many things to do during your day – when are you going to have the time to sit back and be sick?

You have kids, and you know with kids that cuts and scrapes happen, and you hate risking the infection. On the other hand, you don't want to spread chemicals on your child's body when you know that it could cause other side effects – so you feel tied.

What do you do?

If only there was a way you could go all natural with your remedies. If only there was a way you could know without a doubt you were taking care of what needed to be taken care of, but you weren't bringing in harmful side effects while you did it.

If only there was a natural remedy for all the different things you and your children have to deal with during the day.

Or is there?

When you know how to use herbs for your health, you unlock the door to a whole new world. You give yourself the gift of health and healing, and you spare yourself the pain of having to deal with side effects. By taking control of your health through natural remedies, you give yourself the gift of goodness – without anything bad to go along with it.

Have you wanted to get healthy the natural way?

Have you wanted to care for scrapes and bruises without any artificial medication?

You have come to the right place. Let me show you exactly what you need to do to use herbal remedies for a variety of illnesses, and give you perfect control of your life back.

You deserve to be happy and healthy, and with these remedies, you are going to get that very thing.

Let's get started.

Chapter 1 – Herbal Healing

Herbs have been used for thousands of years because of their incredible medicinal properties. Whether you use them as a tea, or you mix them into a salve and apply to the injury itself, you are going to find all kinds of wonderful healing – from the inside out.

Mix up all these different remedies, and enjoy a kind of healing like you never imagined you could have from the natural world. Save on prescriptions. Save time not standing in line at the pharmacy, and save your health with herbs that are meant to heal!

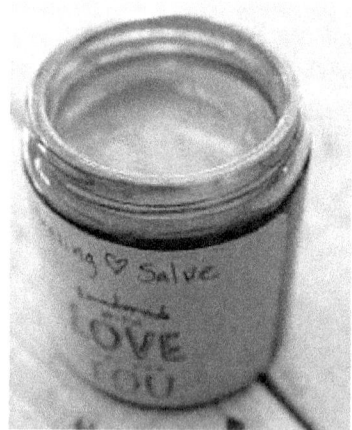

Scratch Sealer

What you will need:

3 tablespoons colloidal silver

8 drops tea tree oil

1/3 cup chopped beeswax

½ cup mango butter

Directions:

Heat 1 cup of water in a stainless steel pan on your stove. Crush the herbs and place them in the boiling water and turn the heat down to a simmer. Allow to simmer for 8 hours.

Strain the herbs out of the water and discard the herbs.

In a double boiler, melt the mango butter and beeswax. Once melted, stir in ½ cup of the herbal infused water. Add the tea tree oil next.

Once all is combined, transfer to another jar to cool.

Apply directly to infected area, and cover with a bandage. Wash the infected area with gentle soap and water and replace with more salve and a clean bandage twice per day.

Infection Fighter

What you will need:

2 tablespoons peppermint leaves

1 tablespoon grated, dried lemon peel

Directions:

Make sure all the herbs you are using are dried and clean. Crush them into smaller pieces and set aside.

Line a tea ball with a paper towel so the finer bits of the herbs do not seep out of the ball as the tea is being prepared. Mix the herbs with 1 tablespoon black tea, and transfer to the ball.

Steep in a mug of hot water for up to 10 minutes, and stir in 1 tablespoon of honey, if desired. Enjoy.

Repeat up to 3 times per day for as long as symptoms persist.

Home Doctor

What you will need:

1 tablespoon chamomile leaves

1 tablespoon licorice leaves

Directions:

Make sure all the herbs you are using are dried and clean. Crush them into smaller pieces and set aside.

Line a tea ball with a paper towel so the finer bits of the herbs do not seep out of the ball as the tea is being prepared. Mix the herbs with 1 tablespoon black tea, and transfer to the ball.

Steep in a mug of hot water for up to 10 minutes, and stir in 1 tablespoon of honey, if desired. Enjoy.

Repeat up to 3 times per day for as long as symptoms persist.

Throat Coat

What you will need:

2 cinnamon sticks, crushed

1 tablespoon lemon zest

1 tablespoon peppermint leaves

Directions:

Make sure all the herbs you are using are dried and clean. Crush them into smaller pieces and set aside.

Line a tea ball with a paper towel so the finer bits of the herbs do not seep out of the ball as the tea is being prepared. Mix the herbs with 1 tablespoon black tea, and transfer to the ball.

Steep in a mug of hot water for up to 10 minutes, and stir in 1 tablespoon of honey, if desired. Enjoy.

Repeat up to 3 times per day for as long as symptoms persist.

Universal Healer

What you will need:

2 tablespoons crushed sage leaves

1 tablespoon slippery elm

Directions:

Make sure all the herbs you are using are dried and clean. Crush them into smaller pieces and set aside.

Line a tea ball with a paper towel so the finer bits of the herbs do not seep out of the ball as the tea is being prepared. Mix the herbs with 1 tablespoon black tea, and transfer to the ball.

Steep in a mug of hot water for up to 10 minutes, and stir in 1 tablespoon of honey, if desired. Enjoy.

Repeat up to 3 times per day for as long as symptoms persist.

Joint Lube

What you will need:

3 tablespoons peppermint leaves

2 tablespoons spearmint leaves

8 drops tea tree oil

1/3 cup chopped beeswax

½ cup mango butter

Directions:

Heat 1 cup of water in a stainless steel pan on your stove. Crush the herbs and place them in the boiling water and turn the heat down to a simmer. Allow to simmer for 8 hours.

Strain the herbs out of the water and discard the herbs.

In a double boiler, melt the mango butter and beeswax. Once melted, stir in ½ cup of the herbal infused water. Add the tea tree oil next.

Once all is combined, transfer to another jar to cool.

Apply directly to infected area, and cover with a bandage. Wash the infected area with gentle soap and water and replace with more salve and a clean bandage twice per day.

Cold and Flu Buster

What you will need:

1 garlic clove

2 tablespoons red root, crushed

Directions:

Make sure all the herbs you are using are dried and clean. Crush them into smaller pieces and set aside.

Line a tea ball with a paper towel so the finer bits of the herbs do not seep out of the ball as the tea is being prepared. Mix the herbs with 1 tablespoon black tea, and transfer to the ball.

Steep in a mug of hot water for up to 10 minutes, and stir in 1 tablespoon of honey, if desired. Enjoy.

Repeat up to 3 times per day for as long as symptoms persist.

Cough Catcher

What you will need:

2 cinnamon sticks, crushed

1 tablespoon crushed dried ginger

1 tablespoon orange zest

Directions:

Make sure all the herbs you are using are dried and clean. Crush them into smaller pieces and set aside.

Line a tea ball with a paper towel so the finer bits of the herbs do not seep out of the ball as the tea is being prepared. Mix the herbs with 1 tablespoon black tea, and transfer to the ball.

Steep in a mug of hot water for up to 10 minutes, and stir in 1 tablespoon of honey, if desired. Enjoy.

Repeat up to 3 times per day for as long as symptoms persist.

All Gain No Pain

What you will need:

1 tablespoon turmeric

2 tablespoons valerian root

8 drops tea tree oil

1/3 cup chopped beeswax

½ cup mango butter

Directions:

Heat 1 cup of water in a stainless steel pan on your stove. Crush the herbs and place them in the boiling water and turn the heat down to a simmer. Allow to simmer for 8 hours.

Strain the herbs out of the water and discard the herbs.

In a double boiler, melt the mango butter and beeswax. Once melted, stir in ½ cup of the herbal infused water. Add the tea tree oil next.

Once all is combined, transfer to another jar to cool.

Apply directly to infected area, and cover with a bandage. Wash the infected area with gentle soap and water and replace with more salve and a clean bandage twice per day.

Against the Grain

What you will need:

3 tablespoons eucommia

8 drops tea tree oil

1/3 cup chopped beeswax

½ cup mango butter

Directions:

Heat 1 cup of water in a stainless steel pan on your stove. Crush the herbs and place them in the boiling water and turn the heat down to a simmer. Allow to simmer for 8 hours.

Strain the herbs out of the water and discard the herbs.

In a double boiler, melt the mango butter and beeswax. Once melted, stir in ½ cup of the herbal infused water. Add the tea tree oil next.

Once all is combined, transfer to another jar to cool.

Apply directly to infected area, and cover with a bandage. Wash the infected area with gentle soap and water and replace with more salve and a clean bandage twice per day.

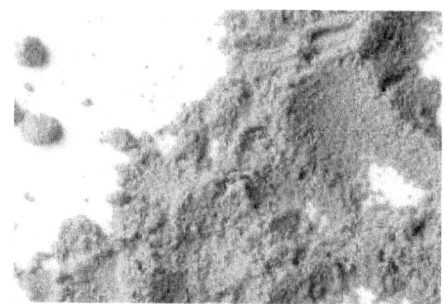

Happy Health

What you will need:

1 tablespoon clean, crushed rose hips

1 tablespoon crushed dried ginger root

Directions:

Make sure all the herbs you are using are dried and clean. Crush them into smaller pieces and set aside.

Line a tea ball with a paper towel so the finer bits of the herbs do not seep out of the ball as the tea is being prepared. Mix the herbs with 1 tablespoon black tea, and transfer to the ball.

Steep in a mug of hot water for up to 10 minutes, and stir in 1 tablespoon of honey, if desired. Enjoy.

Repeat up to 3 times per day for as long as symptoms persist.

Purity

What you will need:

2 tablespoons crushed anise seeds

1 tablespoon crushed peppermint leaves

Directions:

Make sure all the herbs you are using are dried and clean. Crush them into smaller pieces and set aside.

Line a tea ball with a paper towel so the finer bits of the herbs do not seep out of the ball as the tea is being prepared. Mix the herbs with 1 tablespoon black tea, and transfer to the ball.

Steep in a mug of hot water for up to 10 minutes, and stir in 1 tablespoon of honey, if desired. Enjoy.

Repeat up to 3 times per day for as long as symptoms persist.

Breathe Easy

What you will need:

1 teaspoon crushed dried red pepper flakes

3 tablespoons chamomile leaves

Directions:

Make sure all the herbs you are using are dried and clean. Crush them into smaller pieces and set aside.

Line a tea ball with a paper towel so the finer bits of the herbs do not seep out of the ball as the tea is being prepared. Mix the herbs with 1 tablespoon black tea, and transfer to the ball.

Steep in a mug of hot water for up to 10 minutes, and stir in 1 tablespoon of honey, if desired. Enjoy.

Repeat up to 3 times per day for as long as symptoms persist.

This can also be used as a salve and be applied to the patient's neck and chest area. Repeat as often as needed for as long as symptoms persist.

Home Grown Health

What you will need:

1 tablespoon crushed dried burdock

1 tablespoon crushed ginger

Directions:

Make sure all the herbs you are using are dried and clean. Crush them into smaller pieces and set aside.

Line a tea ball with a paper towel so the finer bits of the herbs do not seep out of the ball as the tea is being prepared. Mix the herbs with 1 tablespoon black tea, and transfer to the ball.

Steep in a mug of hot water for up to 10 minutes, and stir in 1 tablespoon of honey, if desired. Enjoy.

Repeat up to 3 times per day for as long as symptoms persist.

Family's Choice

What you will need:

1 tablespoon marshmallow leaves

1 tablespoon licorice leaves

Directions:

Make sure all the herbs you are using are dried and clean. Crush them into smaller pieces and set aside.

Line a tea ball with a paper towel so the finer bits of the herbs do not seep out of the ball as the tea is being prepared. Mix the herbs with 1 tablespoon black tea, and transfer to the ball.

Steep in a mug of hot water for up to 10 minutes, and stir in 1 tablespoon of honey, if desired. Enjoy.

Repeat up to 3 times per day for as long as symptoms persist.

Aches Be Gone

What you will need:

1 tablespoon spearmint leaves

2 tablespoons crushed dried cilantro

8 drops tea tree oil

1/3 cup chopped beeswax

½ cup mango butter

Directions:

Heat 1 cup of water in a stainless steel pan on your stove. Crush the herbs and place them in the boiling water and turn the heat down to a simmer. Allow to simmer for 8 hours.

Strain the herbs out of the water and discard the herbs.

In a double boiler, melt the mango butter and beeswax. Once melted, stir in ½ cup of the herbal infused water. Add the tea tree oil next.

Once all is combined, transfer to another jar to cool.

Apply directly to infected area, and cover with a bandage. Wash the infected area with gentle soap and water and replace with more salve and a clean bandage twice per day.

Going Green

What you will need:

2 tablespoons clean, dried dandelion leaves

1 tablespoon crushed cumin seeds

Directions:

Make sure all the herbs you are using are dried and clean. Crush them into smaller pieces and set aside.

Line a tea ball with a paper towel so the finer bits of the herbs do not seep out of the ball as the tea is being prepared. Mix the herbs with 1 tablespoon black tea, and transfer to the ball.

Steep in a mug of hot water for up to 10 minutes, and stir in 1 tablespoon of honey, if desired. Enjoy.

Repeat up to 3 times per day for as long as symptoms persist.

It's a Health Thing

What you will need:

1 tablespoon dried fennel

2 tablespoons crushed valerian root

Directions:

Make sure all the herbs you are using are dried and clean. Crush them into smaller pieces and set aside.

Line a tea ball with a paper towel so the finer bits of the herbs do not seep out of the ball as the tea is being prepared. Mix the herbs with 1 tablespoon black tea, and transfer to the ball.

Steep in a mug of hot water for up to 10 minutes, and stir in 1 tablespoon of honey, if desired. Enjoy.

Repeat up to 3 times per day for as long as symptoms persist.

Wonder Tea

What you will need:

2 tablespoons dried ginseng

1 tablespoon dried orange zest

Directions:

Make sure all the herbs you are using are dried and clean. Crush them into smaller pieces and set aside.

Line a tea ball with a paper towel so the finer bits of the herbs do not seep out of the ball as the tea is being prepared. Mix the herbs with 1 tablespoon black tea, and transfer to the ball.

Steep in a mug of hot water for up to 10 minutes, and stir in 1 tablespoon of honey, if desired. Enjoy.

Repeat up to 3 times per day for as long as symptoms persist.

Salve Savior

What you will need:

1 tablespoon lavender

1 tablespoon holy basil

8 drops tea tree oil

1/3 cup chopped beeswax

½ cup mango butter

Directions:

Heat 1 cup of water in a stainless steel pan on your stove. Crush the herbs and place them in the boiling water and turn the heat down to a simmer. Allow to simmer for 8 hours.

Strain the herbs out of the water and discard the herbs.

In a double boiler, melt the mango butter and beeswax. Once melted, stir in ½ cup of the herbal infused water. Add the tea tree oil next.

Once all is combined, transfer to another jar to cool.

Apply directly to infected area, and cover with a bandage. Wash the infected area with gentle soap and water and replace with more salve and a clean bandage twice per day.

Better than Medicine

What you will need:

2 tablespoons dried mint leaves

1 tablespoon milk thistle

Directions:

Make sure all the herbs you are using are dried and clean. Crush them into smaller pieces and set aside.

Line a tea ball with a paper towel so the finer bits of the herbs do not seep out of the ball as the tea is being prepared. Mix the herbs with 1 tablespoon black tea, and transfer to the ball.

Steep in a mug of hot water for up to 10 minutes, and stir in 1 tablespoon of honey, if desired. Enjoy.

Repeat up to 3 times per day for as long as symptoms persist.

Sweet Dreams

What you will need:

2 tablespoons lavender leaves

1 tablespoon chamomile leaves

Directions:

Make sure all the herbs you are using are dried and clean. Crush them into smaller pieces and set aside.

Line a tea ball with a paper towel so the finer bits of the herbs do not seep out of the ball as the tea is being prepared. Mix the herbs with 1 tablespoon black tea, and transfer to the ball.

Steep in a mug of hot water for up to 10 minutes, and stir in 1 tablespoon of honey, if desired. Enjoy.

Repeat up to 3 times per day for as long as symptoms persist.

This can also be used as a salve and be applied to the patient's neck and chest area. Repeat as often as needed for as long as symptoms persist.

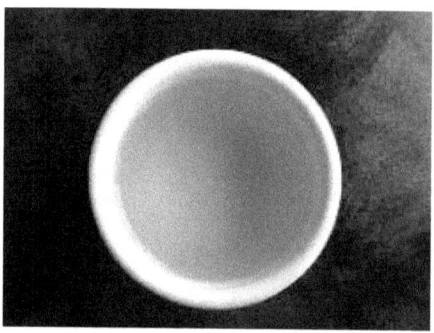

That's the Spot

What you will need:

2 tablespoons oregano

1 tablespoon dried parsley

8 drops tea tree oil

1/3 cup chopped beeswax

½ cup mango butter

Directions:

Heat 1 cup of water in a stainless steel pan on your stove. Crush the herbs and place them in the boiling water and turn the heat down to a simmer. Allow to simmer for 8 hours.

Strain the herbs out of the water and discard the herbs.

In a double boiler, melt the mango butter and beeswax. Once melted, stir in ½ cup of the herbal infused water. Add the tea tree oil next.

Once all is combined, transfer to another jar to cool.

Apply directly to infected area, and cover with a bandage. Wash the infected area with gentle soap and water and replace with more salve and a clean bandage twice per day.

School Days

What you will need:

1 tablespoon lemon mint leaves

1 tablespoon dried lemon zest

Directions:

Make sure all the herbs you are using are dried and clean. Crush them into smaller pieces and set aside.

Line a tea ball with a paper towel so the finer bits of the herbs do not seep out of the ball as the tea is being prepared. Mix the herbs with 1 tablespoon black tea, and transfer to the ball.

Steep in a mug of hot water for up to 10 minutes, and stir in 1 tablespoon of honey, if desired. Enjoy.

Repeat up to 3 times per day for as long as symptoms persist.

24 Hours Later

What you will need:

5 saffron florets

1 tablespoon passionflower leaves

Directions:

Make sure all the herbs you are using are dried and clean. Crush them into smaller pieces and set aside.

Line a tea ball with a paper towel so the finer bits of the herbs do not seep out of the ball as the tea is being prepared. Mix the herbs with 1 tablespoon black tea, and transfer to the ball.

Steep in a mug of hot water for up to 10 minutes, and stir in 1 tablespoon of honey, if desired. Enjoy.

Repeat up to 3 times per day for as long as symptoms persist.

Cool and Clear

What you will need:

1 tablespoon dried mint leaves

1 tablespoon dried peppermint leaves

8 drops tea tree oil

1/3 cup chopped beeswax

½ cup mango butter

Directions:

Heat 1 cup of water in a stainless steel pan on your stove. Crush the herbs and place them in the boiling water and turn the heat down to a simmer. Allow to simmer for 8 hours.

Strain the herbs out of the water and discard the herbs.

In a double boiler, melt the mango butter and beeswax. Once melted, stir in ½ cup of the herbal infused water. Add the tea tree oil next.

Once all is combined, transfer to another jar to cool.

Apply directly to infected area, and cover with a bandage. Wash the infected area with gentle soap and water and replace with more salve and a clean bandage twice per day.

Beautiful

What you will need:

1 tablespoon dried thyme

1 tablespoon dried rosemary

Directions:

Make sure all the herbs you are using are dried and clean. Crush them into smaller pieces and set aside.

Line a tea ball with a paper towel so the finer bits of the herbs do not seep out of the ball as the tea is being prepared. Mix the herbs with 1 tablespoon black tea, and transfer to the ball.

Steep in a mug of hot water for up to 10 minutes, and stir in 1 tablespoon of honey, if desired. Enjoy.

Repeat up to 3 times per day for as long as symptoms persist.

Back on Track

What you will need:

1 tablespoon turmeric

1 tablespoon cloves

Directions:

Make sure all the herbs you are using are dried and clean. Crush them into smaller pieces and set aside.

Line a tea ball with a paper towel so the finer bits of the herbs do not seep out of the ball as the tea is being prepared. Mix the herbs with 1 tablespoon black tea, and transfer to the ball.

Steep in a mug of hot water for up to 10 minutes, and stir in 1 tablespoon of honey, if desired. Enjoy.

Repeat up to 3 times per day for as long as symptoms persist.

What you will need:

1 tablespoon dried rose hips

2 tablespoons rosemary

8 drops tea tree oil

1/3 cup chopped beeswax

½ cup mango butter

Directions:

Heat 1 cup of water in a stainless steel pan on your stove. Crush the herbs and place them in the boiling water and turn the heat down to a simmer. Allow to simmer for 8 hours.

Strain the herbs out of the water and discard the herbs.

In a double boiler, melt the mango butter and beeswax. Once melted, stir in ½ cup of the herbal infused water. Add the tea tree oil next.

Once all is combined, transfer to another jar to cool.

Apply directly to infected area, and cover with a bandage. Wash the infected area with gentle soap and water and replace with more salve and a clean bandage twice per day.

Green Machine

What you will need:

2 tablespoons mint leave

1 teaspoon crushed coriander

Directions:

Make sure all the herbs you are using are dried and clean. Crush them into smaller pieces and set aside.

Line a tea ball with a paper towel so the finer bits of the herbs do not seep out of the ball as the tea is being prepared. Mix the herbs with 1 tablespoon black tea, and transfer to the ball.

Steep in a mug of hot water for up to 10 minutes, and stir in 1 tablespoon of honey, if desired. Enjoy.

Repeat up to 3 times per day for as long as symptoms persist.

Herbal Gurgle

What you will need:

1 tablespoon peppermint leaves

3 tablespoons chamomile leaves

Directions:

Make sure all the herbs you are using are dried and clean. Crush them into smaller pieces and set aside.

Line a tea ball with a paper towel so the finer bits of the herbs do not seep out of the ball as the tea is being prepared. Mix the herbs with 1 tablespoon black tea, and transfer to the ball.

Steep in a mug of hot water for up to 10 minutes, and stir in 1 tablespoon of honey, if desired. Enjoy.

Repeat up to 3 times per day for as long as symptoms persist.

Mother Nature's Favorite Healer

What you will need:

2 teaspoons turmeric

1 teaspoon black pepper

8 drops tea tree oil

1/3 cup chopped beeswax

½ cup mango butter

Directions:

Heat 1 cup of water in a stainless steel pan on your stove. Crush the herbs and place them in the boiling water and turn the heat down to a simmer. Allow to simmer for 8 hours.

Strain the herbs out of the water and discard the herbs.

In a double boiler, melt the mango butter and beeswax. Once melted, stir in ½ cup of the herbal infused water. Add the tea tree oil next.

Once all is combined, transfer to another jar to cool.

Apply directly to infected area, and cover with a bandage. Wash the infected area with gentle soap and water and replace with more salve and a clean bandage twice per day.

It's Scarcely a Scratch

What you will need:

1 tablespoon crushed cinnamon

1 tablespoon crushed garlic

8 drops tea tree oil

1/3 cup chopped beeswax

½ cup mango butter

Directions:

Heat 1 cup of water in a stainless steel pan on your stove. Crush the herbs and place them in the boiling water and turn the heat down to a simmer. Allow to simmer for 8 hours.

Strain the herbs out of the water and discard the herbs.

In a double boiler, melt the mango butter and beeswax. Once melted, stir in ½ cup of the herbal infused water. Add the tea tree oil next.

Once all is combined, transfer to another jar to cool.

Apply directly to infected area, and cover with a bandage. Wash the infected area with gentle soap and water and replace with more salve and a clean bandage twice per day.

When All Else Fails

What you will need:

2 teaspoons ground mustard

1 teaspoon black pepper

Directions:

Make sure all the herbs you are using are dried and clean. Crush them into smaller pieces and set aside.

Line a tea ball with a paper towel so the finer bits of the herbs do not seep out of the ball as the tea is being prepared. Mix the herbs with 1 tablespoon black tea, and transfer to the ball.

Steep in a mug of hot water for up to 10 minutes, and stir in 1 tablespoon of honey, if desired. Enjoy.

Repeat up to 3 times per day for as long as symptoms persist.

Doctor Green

What you will need:

1 teaspoon dried holy basil

1 tablespoon dried thyme

1 teaspoon rosemary leaves

Directions:

Make sure all the herbs you are using are dried and clean. Crush them into smaller pieces and set aside.

Line a tea ball with a paper towel so the finer bits of the herbs do not seep out of the ball as the tea is being prepared. Mix the herbs with 1 tablespoon black tea, and transfer to the ball.

Steep in a mug of hot water for up to 10 minutes, and stir in 1 tablespoon of honey, if desired. Enjoy.

Repeat up to 3 times per day for as long as symptoms persist.

Conclusion

There you have it, everything you need to know to make a variety of your own healing salves and teas – just by using all natural herbs. I hope this book was able to give you the inspiration you need to enjoy natural living, and that you mix up each and every one of these blends for your health today.

You can't put a price on your health, and you certainly don't want to fill your body with all those harmful side effects that you can experience from synthetic medicine. But now, you don't have to.

All these recipes are perfectly safe to use as much as you need to, giving you the power to control your health and enjoy your life while you save money, avoid chemicals, and much, much more.

I hope you feel inspired to change your life with this book, and that it gives you all the rich benefits you have been hoping for.

Happy healing.

FREE Bonus Reminder

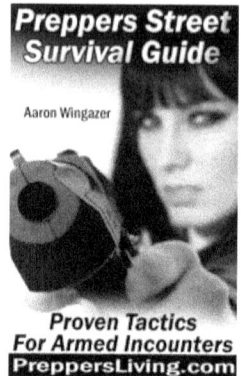

If you have not grabbed it yet, please go ahead and download your special bonus report *"Preppers Street Survival Guide: Proven Tactics For Armed Incounters"*

SimplyClicktheButtonBelow

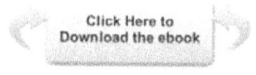

OR **Go to This Page**

http://preppersliving.com/free

BONUS #2: More Free & Discounted Books & Products

Do you want to receive more Free/Discounted Books or Products?

We have a mailing list where we send out our new Books or Products when they go free or with a discount on Amazon. Click on the link below to sign up for Free & Discount Book & Product Promotions.

=> Sign Up for Free & Discount Book & Product Promotions <=

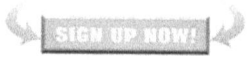

OR Go to this URL

http://zbit.ly/1WBb1Ek